BEEF CATTLE NUTRITION AND FEEDING STRATEGIES

Optimizing Health, Efficiency, And Sustainability In Beef Production

Ethan Harry

Table of Contents

CHAPTER ONE 4

    INTRODUCTION TO BEEF CATTLE NUTRITION 4

    OVERVIEW OF BEEF CATTLE INDUSTRY 9

    IMPORTANCE OF NUTRITION IN BEEF PRODUCTION 13

    NUTRIENT REQUIREMENTS FOR BEEF CATTLE.......................18

    ROLE OF NUTRITION IN ANIMAL HEALTH AND PRODUCTIVITY 22

CHAPTER TWO 28

NUTRITIONAL PHYSIOLOGY OF BEEF CATTLE 28

    DIGESTIVE ANATOMY AND PHYSIOLOGY...............................28

    RUMEN FUNCTION AND MICROBIOLOGY..............................33

    NUTRIENT ABSORPTION AND METABOLISM 38

    FACTORS INFLUENCING DIGESTIVE EFFICIENCY 43

CHAPTER THREE..49

FEEDSTUFFS FOR BEEF CATTLE 49

    FORAGES: TYPES AND NUTRITIONAL VALUE 49

    GRAINS AND CONCENTRATES...53

    BY-PRODUCTS AND ALTERNATIVE FEEDSTUFFS 57

    FEED ADDITIVES AND SUPPLEMENTS 62

CHAPTER FOUR 67

FEEDING STRATEGIES FOR DIFFERENT PRODUCTION STAGES 67

    COW-CALF NUTRITION...67

    NUTRITION FOR GROWING AND FINISHING CATTLE 72

- NUTRITION FOR BREEDING BULLS 76
- SPECIAL CONSIDERATIONS FOR REPLACEMENT HEIFERS 81

CHAPTER FIVE 86

RATION FORMULATION AND FEEDING MANAGEMENT 86

- PRINCIPLES OF RATION FORMULATION 86
- BALANCING RATIONS FOR NUTRIENT NEEDS 91
- FEED MIXING AND DELIVERY METHODS................ 96
- MONITORING AND ADJUSTING FEEDING PROGRAMS 101

CHAPTER SIX 107

HEALTH AND NUTRITION INTERACTIONS ... 107

- NUTRITIONAL DISORDERS AND DEFICIENCIES 107
- ROLE OF NUTRITION IN DISEASE PREVENTION................... 112
- MANAGING STRESS THROUGH NUTRITION 116
- USE OF PROBIOTICS AND PREBIOTICS 121

CHAPTER SEVEN 127

ECONOMIC AND ENVIRONMENTAL CONSIDERATIONS 127

- COST-EFFECTIVE FEEDING STRATEGIES 127
- EVALUATING FEED COSTS AND RETURNS........................... 131
- ENVIRONMENTAL IMPACT OF BEEF CATTLE NUTRITION 136
- SUSTAINABLE FEEDING PRACTICES.. 141

THE END 146

CHAPTER ONE
INTRODUCTION TO BEEF CATTLE NUTRITION

Proper nutrition is fundamental to raising healthy, productive beef cattle. Understanding the nutritional needs of these animals helps farmers ensure their cattle grow efficiently, remain healthy, and produce high-quality beef. Beef cattle nutrition involves providing the right balance of energy, protein, vitamins, minerals, and water. Here's a straightforward guide to understanding the basics of beef cattle nutrition.

Energy

Energy is the most critical component of a beef cow's diet. It fuels all bodily functions, including growth, reproduction, and maintenance. The primary sources of energy in cattle diets are carbohydrates and fats. Carbohydrates come from forages like grass and hay, as well as grains such as corn and barley. Fats are more concentrated energy sources and are sometimes added to cattle feed to boost energy intake.

Protein

Protein is essential for muscle development, growth, and repair. It also plays a crucial role in the production of milk in cows and the overall health of the animal. Protein sources for beef cattle include legumes like alfalfa, soybeans, and commercial protein supplements. Younger, growing cattle require more protein compared to mature cows.

Vitamins and Minerals

Vitamins and minerals are vital for various bodily functions, including bone development, immune function, and reproduction. Important minerals include calcium, phosphorus, magnesium, and potassium. Trace minerals like zinc, copper, and selenium are needed in smaller amounts but are equally important. Vitamins A, D, and E are crucial for maintaining health and preventing deficiencies.

Water

Water is often overlooked but is arguably the most critical nutrient. Cattle require a constant supply of clean, fresh water to regulate body temperature, aid digestion, and support overall health. Water needs vary depending on the animal's size, age, diet, and environmental conditions. On average, an adult cow can drink between 10 to 20 gallons of water per day.

Feeding Strategies

There are different feeding strategies based on the cattle's stage of life and production goals.

1. Forage-Based Diets: Forage, including pasture grass and hay, is the primary component of many beef cattle diets. It provides the necessary fiber for proper digestion and helps maintain rumen health.

2. Grain-Based Diets: These are often used for finishing cattle to increase weight gain and improve meat quality. Grains like corn and barley are high in energy and help cattle gain weight quickly.

3. Supplemental Feeding: Sometimes, additional nutrients are required that are not sufficiently available in the primary feed. Supplements can include protein cakes, mineral blocks, and vitamin mixes.

Ration Balancing

Ration balancing is the process of ensuring that all nutritional requirements are met in the right proportions. This involves calculating the right mix of forages, grains, and supplements to provide a balanced diet that supports growth, reproduction, and health. Farmers often work with nutritionists or use computer programs to create balanced rations tailored to their herd's specific needs.

OVERVIEW OF BEEF CATTLE INDUSTRY

The beef cattle industry is a cornerstone of global agriculture, playing a vital role in producing meat that is a key source of protein for human consumption. This industry is complex and multifaceted, encompassing various stages from breeding to processing. Understanding these segments is crucial for appreciating the industry's structure and its economic significance.

At the foundation of the beef cattle industry are cow-calf operations. These operations focus on breeding cows to produce calves. The process begins with selecting high-quality breeding stock to ensure the health and productivity of the herd. Calves are typically born in the spring or fall and remain with their mothers, grazing on pastureland, until they are weaned at around six to eight months of age. Once weaned, calves are either sold to feedlots or retained for future breeding purposes. Cow-calf operations are fundamental as they supply the initial livestock that fuels the entire beef production chain.

The next critical phase is the feedlot stage, where young cattle are transferred to specialized facilities designed to maximize growth and weight gain. In feedlots, cattle are fed a high-energy diet consisting mainly of grains, such as corn and soybeans, along with forage and supplements. This diet is essential for promoting rapid growth and increasing the animals' weight efficiently. Cattle typically spend several months in feedlots, where they are monitored for health and growth progress. The goal is to achieve an optimal weight and fat composition before they are sent to processing plants for slaughter.

Processing plants represent another key component of the beef cattle industry. These facilities are equipped to handle the slaughter and processing of cattle into various beef cuts and products. The processing phase involves butchering the animals, ensuring food safety standards are met, and preparing the meat for distribution. Beef cuts range from premium steaks and roasts to ground beef and other processed products. These products are then distributed to supermarkets, restaurants, and other food outlets, making their way to consumers' tables.

Beyond the biological and mechanical aspects of production, the beef cattle industry has profound economic implications. It generates significant employment opportunities, ranging from farm labor and feedlot management to roles in transportation, marketing, and retail. The industry's economic impact extends to supporting rural communities where many of these operations are based, contributing to the livelihoods of countless individuals and families. Additionally, the industry stimulates related sectors such as veterinary services, feed production, and agricultural equipment manufacturing.

IMPORTANCE OF NUTRITION IN BEEF PRODUCTION

Nutrition plays a pivotal role in beef production, directly influencing the growth, health, and overall productivity of cattle. Ensuring that cattle receive proper nutrition is essential for their optimal development, efficient attainment of market weight, and the production of high-quality meat. To achieve this, it is critical to understand the specific nutrient requirements of cattle at various stages of their life cycle and to provide a balanced diet that meets these needs.

From birth through to market weight, cattle undergo several distinct stages of growth, each with unique nutritional demands. For example, calves require a diet rich in protein to support rapid growth and development in their early months. As they mature, their dietary needs shift, and they require a diet that supports continued growth while preparing them for the finishing phase, where the focus is on fattening and muscle development.

A balanced diet for cattle typically includes a mix of forages, grains, vitamins, and minerals. Forages, such as grass and hay, are essential for providing fiber, which aids in digestion and overall gut health. Grains, like corn and barley, are crucial energy sources that support growth and weight gain. Vitamins and minerals, though required in smaller quantities, are equally important as they play vital roles in bodily functions, including bone development, immune response, and metabolic processes.

The consequences of inadequate or imbalanced nutrition in cattle can be severe. Poor nutrition can lead to stunted growth, making it difficult for cattle to reach market weight efficiently. It can also increase susceptibility to diseases, as a lack of essential nutrients weakens the immune system. Additionally, cattle that do not receive proper nutrition are more likely to produce lower quality meat, which can affect the profitability of beef production. Issues such as poor marbling, lower meat tenderness, and off-flavors are often linked to nutritional deficiencies.

To avoid these problems, farmers and beef producers must carefully monitor and manage the diets of their cattle. This involves regular assessment of the nutritional content of feed and making necessary adjustments to ensure that all dietary requirements are met. Furthermore, advancements in nutritional science and feed technology have provided producers with tools and knowledge to formulate diets that maximize the efficiency and productivity of their herds.

Moreover, proper nutrition is not only about meeting the immediate needs of the cattle but also about long-term sustainability and animal welfare. By ensuring that cattle are well-nourished, producers can promote healthier animals that are less prone to illness and stress, contributing to more sustainable and ethical farming practices.

NUTRIENT REQUIREMENTS FOR BEEF CATTLE

Beef cattle have specific nutrient requirements that must be met to support their growth, reproduction, and overall health. These requirements encompass several key elements: energy, protein, vitamins, minerals, and water. Each of these nutrients plays a crucial role in maintaining the cattle's well-being and ensuring optimal productivity.

Energy is a fundamental requirement for beef cattle as it supports a wide range of physiological functions, including basic bodily processes, growth, reproduction, and lactation. Energy in a cattle's diet is primarily derived from carbohydrates and fats.

Carbohydrates, found in forages like grasses and hays, and grains like corn and barley, are the primary energy sources. Fats, though present in smaller quantities in most cattle diets, provide a concentrated source of energy. Ensuring that cattle receive adequate energy is critical for maintaining their body condition, promoting efficient growth rates, and supporting milk production in lactating cows.

Protein is another essential nutrient, vital for muscle development, repair, and overall growth. Proteins are composed of amino acids, some of which are essential and must be supplied through the diet because cattle cannot synthesize them. Sources of protein for beef cattle include forages, grains, and supplemental feeds like soybean meal or alfalfa. Adequate protein intake is particularly important for young, growing cattle and for cows during gestation and lactation. Without sufficient protein, cattle can experience stunted growth, poor muscle development, and decreased reproductive performance.

Vitamins and minerals are required in smaller amounts compared to energy and protein but are nonetheless crucial for various bodily functions. Vitamins such as A, D, and E play significant roles in vision, bone health, and immune function, respectively. Minerals like calcium, phosphorus, and magnesium are essential for bone development, metabolic processes, and nerve function. Trace minerals, including zinc, copper, and selenium, are also important despite being required in minute quantities. They support immune function, reproductive health, and enzyme activities. For instance, calcium and phosphorus are critical for skeletal health and milk production, while selenium and vitamin E work together to protect cells from oxidative damage.

Water is perhaps the most vital nutrient for beef cattle. It is essential for digestion, nutrient absorption, and temperature regulation. Water intake can significantly impact cattle health and productivity. Factors such as temperature, diet, and physiological state influence water requirements. Cattle consuming high-fiber diets or experiencing hot weather will require more water. Moreover, water quality is just as important as quantity. Contaminated or poor-quality water can lead to health issues and reduced feed intake, adversely affecting overall performance.

ROLE OF NUTRITION IN ANIMAL HEALTH AND PRODUCTIVITY

Nutrition plays an integral role in the health and productivity of beef cattle, significantly impacting their overall well-being and the economic efficiency of beef production. A well-balanced diet is essential for maintaining the health of cattle by supporting their immune system. A robust immune system enables cattle to better resist diseases and recover from illnesses more swiftly. This aspect of nutrition is particularly crucial for young, growing animals, as well as for pregnant or lactating cows, which have higher nutritional requirements.

For young animals, adequate nutrition is vital for growth and development. Nutrients such as proteins, vitamins, and minerals are necessary for building muscle, bone, and other tissues. Proper growth during the early stages of life ensures that cattle reach their genetic potential for size and weight, which is a key factor in beef production. For pregnant and lactating cows, nutrition is equally critical. These animals need sufficient nutrients to support the development of the fetus and to produce milk of adequate quality and quantity for the newborn calf. Inadequate nutrition during these stages can lead to poor fetal development, lower birth weights, and reduced milk production, all of which can have long-term negative effects on the productivity and profitability of the herd.

Reproductive performance in beef cattle is also closely linked to their nutritional status. Well-nourished cows are more likely to conceive, carry pregnancies to term, and give birth to healthy calves. Energy, protein, and mineral balance in the diet influence reproductive hormones and fertility rates. For instance, deficiencies in key nutrients can lead to irregular estrous cycles, poor conception rates, and increased incidences of calving difficulties. This not only affects the immediate reproductive success but also impacts the long-term sustainability of the herd. Additionally, proper nutrition enhances feed efficiency, which is the amount of feed required to produce a certain amount of meat. Efficient feed utilization is a crucial economic factor for beef producers, as it directly influences feeding costs and return on investment. Cattle that are fed a balanced diet convert feed into body mass more effectively, leading to faster growth rates and shorter time to market. This efficiency not only reduces the cost of feed per unit of meat produced but also improves the overall profitability of beef production.

Conversely, poor nutrition can lead to a multitude of health issues. Metabolic disorders such as ketosis and acidosis, weakened immune function, and poor growth rates are common problems associated with inadequate or imbalanced diets. These health issues not only diminish the well-being of the cattle but also lead to increased veterinary costs, higher mortality rates, and lower overall productivity. For instance, cattle suffering from nutritional deficiencies are more susceptible to infections, experience slower recovery times, and have lower rates of weight gain, all of which reduce the economic viability of the beef production operation.

CHAPTER TWO

NUTRITIONAL PHYSIOLOGY OF BEEF CATTLE

DIGESTIVE ANATOMY AND PHYSIOLOGY

Beef cattle possess a remarkable digestive system known as a ruminant system, finely tuned to effectively process tough, fibrous plant materials. This specialized anatomy consists of several interconnected organs: the mouth, esophagus, stomach, small intestine, and large intestine. Each plays a crucial role in the overall digestive process, ensuring that cattle derive maximum nutrition from their diet.

At the forefront of this digestive marvel is the stomach, divided into four distinct compartments: the rumen, reticulum, omasum, and abomasum. Each compartment serves a unique purpose in the complex process of breaking down plant material and extracting nutrients.

The rumen stands as the largest compartment, occupying a significant portion of the abdominal cavity in cattle. Here, an intricate ecosystem of microorganisms thrives, crucial for the initial breakdown of fibrous plant material through fermentation. This process yields volatile fatty acids, which serve as a primary energy source for the animal. The rumen's environment is highly specialized, maintaining optimal conditions for the microbial community to thrive and efficiently digest cellulose and other complex carbohydrates.

Adjacent to the rumen is the reticulum, often referred to as the "honeycomb" due to its distinctive structure. Functionally, the reticulum works closely with the rumen, aiding in the fermentation process and facilitating the regurgitation of partially digested food for further chewing. This regurgitated cud undergoes extensive rechewing to further break down plant fibers and enhance digestion before it continues its journey through the digestive tract.

Following the rumen and reticulum, the partially digested food enters the omasum. This compartment acts as a filtration system, primarily absorbing water and essential nutrients from the digesta before passing it along to the next stage of digestion. The omasum's role in water absorption helps maintain fluid balance within the animal and ensures efficient nutrient extraction from the digesta.

Finally, the abomasum functions similarly to the monogastric stomach found in non-ruminant animals, including humans. Often referred to as the "true stomach" of ruminants, the abomasum secretes gastric juices containing digestive enzymes such as pepsin and hydrochloric acid. These enzymes play a crucial role in breaking down proteins into smaller peptides and amino acids, facilitating their absorption in the small intestine. This compartment represents the final stage of enzymatic digestion before the nutrients are absorbed and utilized by the animal's body for growth, maintenance, and energy.

Together, these four compartments form a highly efficient digestive system tailored to the dietary needs of beef cattle. By sequentially processing and fermenting fibrous plant materials, cattle can derive essential nutrients and energy from feed that would be indigestible to many other animals. This adaptation not only highlights the evolutionary advantages of ruminant physiology but also underscores the importance of efficient nutrient utilization in agricultural practices. Understanding and optimizing this digestive process are crucial for ensuring the health, productivity, and sustainability of beef cattle production systems worldwide.

RUMEN FUNCTION AND MICROBIOLOGY

The rumen, an essential component of the digestive system in ruminant animals such as cattle, functions as a dynamic fermentation chamber where a complex community of microorganisms collaborates to break down fibrous plant material. This microbial ecosystem within the rumen is comprised primarily of bacteria, protozoa, and fungi, each playing distinct roles crucial to the digestive processes that sustain these animals.

Bacteria are the predominant inhabitants of the rumen, responsible for a myriad of metabolic activities. One of their primary roles is the breakdown of complex carbohydrates, such as cellulose and hemicellulose, which constitute the bulk of plant cell walls. These carbohydrates are formidable barriers to digestion for cattle themselves due to the lack of specific enzymes required to cleave their bonds effectively. Bacteria produce a range of enzymes that can hydrolyze these complex polysaccharides into simpler sugars like glucose, which can then be absorbed by the host animal as a source of energy. Furthermore, bacteria also metabolize proteins, breaking them down into amino acids and other nitrogenous compounds that are subsequently utilized by both the microbes themselves and the ruminant.

Protozoa, another crucial group of rumen microbes, contribute significantly to the digestive process by aiding in the breakdown of starches and proteins. They possess specialized enzymes that can degrade starch molecules, complementing the bacterial activity in carbohydrate digestion. Moreover, protozoa participate in a form of microbial predation, consuming bacteria within the rumen. This predation helps regulate the bacterial population, maintaining a balanced microbial ecosystem essential for efficient digestion. By preying on bacteria, protozoa play a pivotal role in controlling microbial diversity and ensuring that no single microbial species dominates the ruminal environment to the detriment of overall digestion efficiency.

Fungi also play a vital role in the rumen ecosystem, particularly in the degradation of tough plant fibers. These fibers, such as lignin and cellulose, are highly resistant to enzymatic degradation. However, certain fungal species within the rumen produce enzymes known as cellulases and ligninases, which can break down these recalcitrant compounds. By enzymatically degrading tough fibers, fungi facilitate easier access to the cellulose and hemicellulose components for bacterial degradation. This synergistic relationship between fungi and bacteria underscores the complexity and efficiency of the ruminal microbial community in converting plant material into nutrients that can be utilized by the host animal.

Collectively, the rumen microbiota forms a finely tuned ecosystem where bacteria, protozoa, and fungi collaborate synergistically to overcome the challenges posed by the complex plant materials that constitute the ruminant diet. This microbial consortium not only enables the efficient breakdown of fibrous plant materials but also enhances the nutritional value derived from these otherwise indigestible components. The intricate interactions among these microbial groups highlight the remarkable adaptation of ruminants to utilize plant biomass effectively, contributing significantly to their ability to thrive on a diet predominantly composed of fibrous plant material.

NUTRIENT ABSORPTION AND METABOLISM

After undergoing initial digestion in the rumen, the digesta progresses through the subsequent compartments of the stomach before reaching the intestines, where further crucial processes of digestion and nutrient absorption take place.

The small intestine serves as the principal site for nutrient absorption in ruminants. This organ plays a pivotal role in the digestive process by facilitating the breakdown of complex nutrients into forms that can be readily absorbed into the bloodstream. Here, specialized enzymes continue the digestion of proteins into amino acids, fats into fatty acids, and carbohydrates into simple sugars. This enzymatic breakdown is essential as it prepares these nutrients for absorption across the intestinal wall, where they enter the bloodstream and are transported throughout the body to support various physiological functions and metabolic processes.

The absorption of nutrients in the small intestine is a highly efficient process due to its extensive surface area, which is lined with millions of tiny, finger-like projections called villi and microvilli. These structures significantly increase the absorptive surface area, allowing for maximal uptake of nutrients from the digesta passing through the intestinal lumen. The villi are richly supplied with blood vessels and lymphatic vessels (lacteals) that transport absorbed nutrients away from the intestine to be utilized by cells or stored for future energy needs.

In contrast, the large intestine primarily functions to absorb water and certain minerals from the remaining indigestible materials that pass through from the small intestine. While fermentation continues in the large intestine, its role in nutrient absorption is secondary compared to the small intestine and rumen. The microbial population present in the large intestine assists in breaking down remaining fibrous materials and produces certain vitamins, such as vitamin K and some B vitamins, which are absorbed by the host animal.

The process of fermentation in the large intestine differs from that in the rumen in several key aspects. It occurs to a lesser extent and involves different microbial populations adapted to the environment of the large intestine, which is less conducive to extensive fermentation compared to the rumen's anaerobic conditions. The fermentation products in the large intestine, such as volatile fatty acids, contribute to the overall energy metabolism of the animal, albeit to a lesser degree compared to the fermentation occurring in the rumen.

Overall, the journey of digesta through the ruminant digestive system highlights the specialized adaptations of each digestive compartment to maximize the extraction and utilization of nutrients from plant-based diets. From initial digestion in the rumen to final absorption in the small and large intestines, each stage plays a crucial role in ensuring that ruminants efficiently convert plant materials into usable energy and nutrients necessary for growth, maintenance, and production purposes. Understanding these processes is essential for optimizing ruminant nutrition and health, ensuring that dietary needs are met to support the animal's overall well-being and productivity.

FACTORS INFLUENCING DIGESTIVE EFFICIENCY

Factors influencing the efficiency of digestion and nutrient absorption in beef cattle are multifaceted, encompassing diet composition, feed processing methods, feeding management practices, animal health status, and water availability. Each of these elements plays a crucial role in ensuring optimal digestive efficiency and nutrient utilization in cattle farming.

Diet Composition: The composition of a cattle diet profoundly impacts digestive processes. Different types and qualities of feed affect how efficiently nutrients are absorbed. High-fiber diets, typical of forage-based feeding, require extensive microbial fermentation in the rumen to break down complex carbohydrates. This fermentation process yields volatile fatty acids (VFAs), which are a primary energy source for cattle. On the other hand, diets rich in starch from grains are more readily digestible but require careful management to prevent disruptions in the rumen microbial population. Balancing these components ensures cattle receive necessary nutrients while maintaining rumen health.

Feed Processing: Physical processing techniques such as grinding or pelleting can significantly enhance feed digestibility. By breaking down plant cell walls, these methods increase the surface area available for microbial action and enzymatic breakdown in the digestive tract. This improves nutrient accessibility, especially in fibrous feeds like hay or silage. Properly processed feed promotes efficient digestion and absorption of essential nutrients, contributing to overall cattle health and performance.

Feeding Management: Effective feeding management practices are critical for maintaining digestive efficiency. Consistency in feed quality and delivery schedules helps stabilize the rumen environment, supporting optimal microbial activity. Abrupt changes in diet can disrupt the balance of rumen microorganisms, leading to digestive upsets and reduced nutrient absorption. Therefore, gradual transitions between feed types and adherence to regular feeding times are essential to support healthy digestion in cattle.

Animal Health: The health status of cattle directly influences their ability to digest and absorb nutrients efficiently. Healthy animals have robust immune systems and well-functioning digestive tracts, which support effective nutrient utilization. Conversely, diseases, parasitic infections, and stressful conditions compromise digestive function, reducing feed intake and nutrient absorption efficiency. Regular health monitoring and prompt veterinary care are essential to identify and address potential health issues that could impact cattle digestion and overall performance.

Water Availability: Adequate water intake is vital for proper digestion and nutrient transport in cattle. Water facilitates the breakdown and absorption of nutrients in the digestive tract and helps regulate body temperature. Dehydration can lead to reduced feed intake and impaired digestion, affecting overall cattle health and productivity. Access to clean, fresh water is therefore crucial to ensure cattle can effectively utilize the nutrients from their diet and maintain optimal digestive function.

CHAPTER THREE
FEEDSTUFFS FOR BEEF CATTLE
FORAGES: TYPES AND NUTRITIONAL VALUE

Forages play a pivotal role in the diet and nutrition of beef cattle, serving as primary sources of fiber, energy, and essential nutrients in their natural grazing environments. Understanding the types and nutritional contributions of forages is crucial for optimizing cattle health and productivity.

Grasses constitute a significant portion of cattle diets, encompassing diverse species such as bermudagrass, fescue, and ryegrass. These grasses provide substantial bulk and fiber, which are essential for proper digestion and rumen function in cattle. The nutritional content of grasses varies significantly with factors like maturity and growing conditions. Young, actively growing grass tends to be higher in protein and energy compared to mature grass, which is higher in fiber and lignin. Management practices such as rotational grazing can help maintain optimal nutrient levels by ensuring cattle have access to high-quality forage. Legumes such as alfalfa and clover are another important category of forages. These plants are renowned for their higher protein content compared to grasses, making them valuable supplements in cattle diets. Legumes also contribute to soil fertility through symbiotic relationships with nitrogen-fixing bacteria, which enrich the soil with nitrogen. This dual benefit of providing protein-rich forage for cattle while enhancing soil nutrient levels underscores the ecological and nutritional importance of legumes in sustainable beef production systems.

Silages represent a preserved form of forage critical for sustaining cattle through periods of scarcity such as winter months. Silages like corn silage and haylage are produced through anaerobic fermentation, which preserves much of their nutritional value. This preservation method ensures that cattle have access to consistent, high-quality forage even when fresh grazing options are limited. Corn silage, for example, retains its energy content and provides a source of fermentable carbohydrates that support microbial activity in the rumen, thereby aiding in efficient digestion and nutrient utilization by cattle.

Each type of forage contributes distinctively to the nutritional profile of cattle diets. Grasses supply the bulk and structural components necessary for effective rumination and digestive health. Legumes enhance protein intake and soil fertility, promoting sustainable agriculture practices. Silages provide a reliable source of preserved forage during seasons of scarcity, ensuring continuous nutrition for cattle.

GRAINS AND CONCENTRATES

Grains and concentrates play a crucial role in the nutritional management of beef cattle, providing energy-dense supplements to complement forage-based diets and promote efficient growth. These feedstuffs, including corn, barley, and oats, are integral components of modern beef cattle feeding strategies, tailored to meet the specific nutritional needs at different stages of production.

Corn stands out prominently among grains used in beef cattle diets due to its exceptionally high energy content. It serves as a primary source of rapidly fermentable carbohydrates in the rumen, converting into readily available energy that supports both growth and maintenance requirements of cattle. This energy-dense nature makes corn particularly valuable in finishing diets, where the goal is to achieve rapid weight gain and efficient muscle development prior to market readiness.

Barley, another widely utilized grain, offers a balanced nutritional profile characterized by a higher protein content compared to corn. This makes it particularly beneficial in diets where protein supplementation is necessary to support growth and muscle development. Barley's ability to provide sustained energy release, coupled with its relatively high digestibility, enhances its suitability for feeding programs aimed at optimizing cattle performance during various production phases.

In contrast, oats, while also used in beef cattle diets, offer a different nutritional profile compared to corn and barley. Oats are notable for their higher fiber content, which contributes to a more balanced energy release over time. This characteristic makes oats a preferred choice in diets where a slower, more sustained energy source is desired, promoting steady growth and supporting digestive health in cattle.

Concentrates, generally defined by their higher concentrations of energy and protein relative to forages, play a crucial role in achieving specific production goals, such as rapid growth and efficient feed conversion. These feedstuffs are strategically incorporated into cattle diets to supplement the nutrients provided by forages, ensuring that the nutritional requirements for growth, maintenance, and reproductive functions are adequately met.

In practical feeding scenarios, the selection and formulation of grain and concentrate blends are meticulously planned to optimize nutrient utilization and cost-effectiveness while addressing the nutritional demands of beef cattle at different stages of their lifecycle. This involves balancing energy, protein, fiber, and other essential nutrients to achieve desired growth rates, muscle development, and overall herd health.

Moreover, the digestibility and fermentability of these grains and concentrates in the rumen are critical considerations in formulating diets that promote efficient feed utilization and minimize digestive disorders. The ability of these feedstuffs to support rumen microbial activity and maintain a healthy digestive environment contributes significantly to the overall well-being and performance of beef cattle.

BY-PRODUCTS AND ALTERNATIVE FEEDSTUFFS

By-products and alternative feedstuffs play a crucial role in modern beef cattle diets by providing economical sources of nutrients that can supplement or even replace traditional feed ingredients. These alternative feedstuffs offer diverse nutritional benefits, contributing to both the economic efficiency and the nutritional balance of beef cattle rations. One prominent example of such feedstuffs is distillers' grains, a by-product derived from ethanol production. This feedstuff is highly valued for its rich content of protein and energy, making it an effective substitute for grains in feedlot diets. By incorporating distillers' grains, producers can achieve significant cost savings while maintaining the necessary nutritional standards for beef cattle.

Cottonseed meal represents another important alternative feedstuff. It is a high-protein feed made from cottonseed following oil extraction. Despite its nutritional benefits, caution must be exercised due to the presence of gossypol, a toxic compound for ruminants. Proper management practices are essential to mitigate any potential risks associated with gossypol, ensuring the safe and effective utilization of cottonseed meal in cattle diets.

Citrus pulp, a by-product from the citrus juice extraction process, serves as an excellent source of energy and fiber. Beyond its nutritional contributions, citrus pulp enhances diet palatability and increases energy density, making it a favorable choice for beef cattle rations.

Its inclusion in diets helps to maintain optimal energy levels and digestive health in cattle.

Beet pulp, derived from sugar beet processing, is renowned for its high fiber content. This by-product is valued for its digestible fiber and energy contributions to cattle diets. By incorporating beet pulp, producers can effectively enhance the fiber profile of rations, supporting healthy digestion and overall cattle well-being.

In addition to these specific by-products, various alternative protein sources play a pivotal role in beef cattle nutrition. Soybean meal, canola meal, and sunflower meal are recognized for their high-quality protein content. These protein sources are commonly utilized to supplement protein derived from forages, ensuring that cattle receive the essential amino acids necessary for growth, maintenance, and reproduction. The strategic use of these alternative feedstuffs not only diversifies the nutrient profile of beef cattle diets but also offers economic advantages by potentially reducing feed costs. Producers can optimize feed formulations based on the availability and pricing of these by-products and alternative sources, thereby enhancing overall operational efficiency.

Moreover, incorporating these feedstuffs promotes sustainability within the beef cattle industry by utilizing agricultural by-products that might otherwise go to waste. This practice aligns with broader efforts to minimize environmental impact and maximize resource efficiency in livestock production systems.

FEED ADDITIVES AND SUPPLEMENTS

Feed additives and supplements play a crucial role in modern cattle farming by enhancing nutrition, improving feed efficiency, and maintaining overall health. These additives encompass a variety of substances designed to address specific nutritional deficiencies or optimize physiological processes in cattle.

Mineral Supplements are vital components of cattle diets, providing essential minerals such as calcium, phosphorus, magnesium, and trace minerals like zinc, copper, and selenium. These minerals are crucial for bone development, nerve function, muscle contraction, and overall metabolic processes. Insufficient intake of minerals can lead to deficiencies, affecting growth rates, reproductive performance, and susceptibility to diseases. Farmers often supplement feed with mineral blocks or premixed mineral powders to ensure cattle receive adequate amounts based on their age, reproductive status, and environmental conditions.

Vitamin Supplements are another essential category, including vitamins A,

D, E, and various B-complex vitamins. Vitamins play pivotal roles in maintaining immune function, vision, skin health, and reproductive efficiency. For example, vitamin A is essential for vision and immune function, while vitamin D aids in calcium absorption and bone health. Vitamin E acts as an antioxidant, protecting cells from oxidative damage, and the B-complex vitamins are involved in energy metabolism and nervous system function. Supplementing these vitamins ensures that cattle receive consistent levels necessary for optimal health and performance.

Ionophores are feed additives that modify rumen fermentation patterns, improving feed efficiency and reducing methane production. Common ionophores used in cattle farming include monensin and lasalocid. These compounds alter microbial activity in the rumen, increasing the efficiency with which cattle convert feed into energy and growth. This not only enhances overall feed utilization but also reduces the environmental impact associated with methane emissions from livestock.

Antibiotics are sometimes used judiciously in cattle farming to prevent and treat diseases, thereby promoting growth and improving feed efficiency. While their primary role is to combat bacterial infections, antibiotics also have secondary benefits in enhancing nutrient absorption and minimizing losses due to subclinical infections. However, their use is carefully regulated to mitigate the development of antibiotic resistance and ensure food safety standards are upheld.

Each of these feed additives and supplements serves a specific purpose in cattle nutrition and management. They are integrated into feeding programs based on nutritional assessments, production goals, and veterinary recommendations. By carefully balancing these additives, farmers can optimize the health, growth, and productivity of their cattle herds while adhering to sustainable farming practices.

CHAPTER FOUR

FEEDING STRATEGIES FOR DIFFERENT PRODUCTION STAGES

COW-CALF NUTRITION

Cow-calf operations are dedicated to the production of robust calves destined for either beef production or as replacement heifers. The nutritional demands placed on cows vary significantly throughout their reproductive cycle, necessitating careful management to ensure both maternal health and optimal calf development.

Gestation Phase Nutrition:

During gestation, cows undergo a crucial period where nutritional requirements play a pivotal role in supporting fetal growth and development. A balanced diet is paramount, ensuring adequate levels of protein, energy, vitamins, and minerals, with particular emphasis on calcium and phosphorus. These nutrients are essential for skeletal formation and overall fetal health.

Protein is vital as it supports tissue development in the fetus, while energy ensures the cow maintains a healthy weight and provides ample resources for both herself and the growing calf. Vitamins, including A, D, and E, are critical for various metabolic processes and immune function, ensuring both cow and calf remain healthy throughout the gestation period. Minerals like calcium and phosphorus are necessary for bone development and to prevent deficiencies that could affect both the cow and the calf.

Nutritional management strategies during gestation aim to optimize cow health to facilitate a strong and healthy calf at birth. Monitoring body condition scores and adjusting feed rations accordingly is common practice to ensure cows maintain an appropriate weight and condition throughout pregnancy.

Lactation Phase Nutrition:

Following calving, cows transition into the lactation phase, a period marked by increased nutritional demands to support milk production and continued calf growth. The quality of the diet becomes paramount, with a focus on providing sufficient energy and protein to sustain lactation while promoting calf growth.

Energy requirements skyrocket during lactation as cows expend significant energy producing milk. Adequate dietary energy prevents weight loss in the cow and ensures she can meet the demands of both milk production and her own maintenance. Protein is crucial for milk synthesis and to support the growth of the calf, particularly during the first few months of life when rapid growth occurs.

Supplementation may be necessary during lactation to prevent deficiencies and metabolic disorders such as milk fever, which can occur due to the sudden increase in calcium demand for milk production. Magnesium supplementation may also be considered to maintain proper metabolic function in lactating cows.

Balancing these nutritional needs requires careful consideration of both the quantity and quality of feed provided to lactating cows. Diets are often formulated with high-quality forages and grains to meet these heightened requirements effectively. Monitoring milk production, calf growth rates, and the overall health of the cow helps ensure nutritional strategies are effective throughout the lactation phase.

NUTRITION FOR GROWING AND FINISHING CATTLE

Nutrition plays a crucial role in the growth and development of cattle, especially during the phases of growth and finishing. These stages demand specific dietary strategies to ensure optimal muscle development, efficient weight gain, and overall health.

Growing Phase: During the growing phase, which encompasses the early stages of cattle development, the primary objective is to support skeletal and muscle growth. Young cattle require diets rich in both protein and energy to facilitate these processes effectively. The foundation of their diet often consists of forages supplemented with grains or protein-rich concentrates. Forages provide essential roughage and some nutrients, while grains contribute concentrated energy and additional protein.

Protein is particularly vital during this stage as it aids in the formation of muscle tissue. Cattle convert dietary protein into amino acids, which are the building blocks for muscle growth and repair. Alongside protein, energy sources like grains (such as corn or barley) are crucial for meeting the high metabolic demands of growth. These grains provide carbohydrates that supply the energy needed for cellular functions and overall body maintenance. Mineral supplementation is another critical aspect of the growing phase.

Minerals like calcium and phosphorus are essential for bone development and skeletal strength. Additionally, minerals such as copper, zinc, and selenium play roles in various metabolic processes and immune function, ensuring overall health and growth.

Finishing Phase: As cattle approach market weight, they enter the finishing phase, where the emphasis shifts towards maximizing lean muscle growth and achieving desirable carcass quality, including marbling. Finishing diets are specifically formulated to rapidly increase weight while enhancing meat quality attributes.

The cornerstone of finishing diets is energy. Grains, particularly corn and barley, are primary sources of energy due to their high starch content. Starches in grains are efficiently converted into glucose, providing the energy needed for rapid growth and weight gain. This phase aims to balance energy intake with protein levels to optimize growth rates and feed efficiency.

Protein remains crucial during finishing as well, albeit in slightly different proportions compared to the growing phase. High-quality protein sources, often derived from grains and protein concentrates, ensure that cattle maintain muscle mass and continue to develop lean meat.

Mineral supplementation continues to be essential during the finishing phase. Adequate levels of minerals and vitamins, including vitamin E for antioxidant protection and selenium for immune function, are crucial to support overall health and enhance meat quality.

NUTRITION FOR BREEDING BULLS

Nutrition plays a crucial role in the reproductive performance, health, and longevity of breeding bulls. Properly managing their diet ensures they maintain optimal condition and support successful breeding outcomes.

Energy and Protein Requirements:

Breeding bulls have elevated energy needs due to their reproductive activities. Adequate energy intake is essential for maintaining body condition and supporting overall health. Typically, diets for breeding bulls are supplemented with grains or protein concentrates to meet these high energy demands. These supplements help ensure bulls receive sufficient calories to support their metabolic functions, including sperm production and activity. Alongside energy, high-quality protein is vital for bulls. Protein serves as the building block for tissues and is particularly important for the production of sperm cells. Bulls require a balanced supply of amino acids, the building blocks of protein, to support their reproductive processes effectively.

Vitamins and Minerals:

Key vitamins and minerals play critical roles in the reproductive health of breeding bulls. Vitamin A is essential for the development and maintenance of epithelial tissues, including those within the reproductive tract. Vitamin D aids in calcium absorption and bone health, crucial for maintaining structural integrity and overall health. Vitamin E functions as an antioxidant, protecting cells from oxidative stress, which can impact sperm quality.

Minerals such as selenium and zinc are also pivotal. Selenium supports sperm motility and function, playing a vital role in reproductive success. Zinc is necessary for the synthesis of DNA and RNA, fundamental processes in cell division and sperm production. These micronutrients are often supplemented in bull diets to ensure adequate levels necessary for optimal reproductive performance.

Body Condition Score (BCS):

Maintaining an optimal body condition score (BCS) is paramount for breeding success in bulls. A BCS scale typically ranges from 1 to 9, with scores around 5 being ideal for most breeding bulls. Bulls with a BCS that is too high (overweight) or too low (underweight) may experience reduced fertility. Overweight bulls may have decreased libido and increased difficulty mounting females, while underweight bulls may have reduced sperm quality and production.

Regular assessment and management of body condition involve adjusting diet and exercise regimens as needed to maintain bulls within the optimal BCS range. This proactive approach helps prevent reproductive issues associated with extremes in body condition.

Overall Management:

Nutritional management of breeding bulls requires a holistic approach, considering not only the quantity of nutrients but also their quality and balance. Diets should be formulated based on the specific requirements of each bull, considering factors such as age, breed, and reproductive status. Regular veterinary assessments and monitoring of reproductive performance are essential to adjust nutritional strategies as bulls progress through different stages of their reproductive lifespan.

SPECIAL CONSIDERATIONS FOR REPLACEMENT HEIFERS

Ensuring the optimal growth and development of replacement heifers is paramount for securing the future reproductive success of a cattle herd. These young females represent the next generation of breeding stock, requiring meticulous nutritional management from birth through maturity.

Growth and Development

From the moment a heifer is born, her nutritional journey begins. The goal is to achieve adequate growth rates so that she reaches the target breeding weight by around 15 to 18 months of age. This milestone ensures she can conceive and calve at an appropriate age, contributing to the herd's productivity. Central to this growth is a diet rich in proteins and energy, which support skeletal development and overall body growth. These nutrients are crucial during the formative stages when the heifer's body is rapidly developing, laying the foundation for future reproductive health.

Reproductive Health

Nutrition plays a pivotal role in a heifer's reproductive health. Proper development of the reproductive system, including the onset of puberty and regular estrous cycles, hinges on receiving adequate nutrition. Nutrients such as proteins, minerals, and vitamins influence hormone production and follicular development. Insufficient nutrition can delay puberty, prolonging the time it takes for the heifer to become reproductively active. Conversely, an optimally balanced diet ensures that she reaches puberty at the appropriate age, setting the stage for timely breeding and conception.

Mineral Supplementation

In addition to protein and energy, minerals are critical for the skeletal development of replacement heifers. Calcium and phosphorus are particularly essential, as they support bone formation and prevent deficiencies that could impair future productivity. Ensuring these minerals are present in the heifer's diet at adequate levels is crucial throughout her growth phase. Deficiencies can lead to skeletal abnormalities or weakened bones, impacting her ability to carry a calf to term and her long-term health as a breeding female.

Nutritional Management

Managing the diet of replacement heifers requires a delicate balance. It is essential to avoid excessive growth rates, which can lead to metabolic issues or skeletal disorders. On the other hand, undernutrition can stunt growth and delay reproductive maturity, ultimately reducing the heifer's lifetime productivity. Regular monitoring of body weight, body condition score (BCS), and reproductive maturity guides nutritional decisions. Adjustments in diet composition and feeding strategies ensure that each heifer progresses towards her target weight and reproductive readiness at the appropriate pace.

CHAPTER FIVE

RATION FORMULATION AND FEEDING MANAGEMENT

PRINCIPLES OF RATION FORMULATION

Ration formulation is a critical process in the management of beef cattle, aiming to create diets that precisely meet their nutritional needs across various stages of production. This methodical approach ensures optimal health, growth, and reproduction, while also considering factors like environmental conditions and economic feasibility.

Central to ration formulation is a deep understanding of the specific nutrient requirements of cattle. These requirements vary significantly depending on factors such as age, weight, and physiological state (e.g., growth, lactation). For instance, growing calves have different nutritional needs compared to lactating cows or bulls intended for breeding. By accurately assessing these needs, nutritionists can tailor diets that provide adequate energy, protein, vitamins, and minerals essential for maintaining health and supporting productive functions.

Selecting appropriate feed ingredients is another cornerstone of effective ration formulation. Feedstuffs such as forages, grains, by-products, and supplements are chosen based on their nutrient profiles, availability, and cost-effectiveness. For example, high-quality forages may be preferred for their fiber content and digestibility, while grains and protein supplements can be added to meet specific protein and energy requirements. Balancing these ingredients ensures that the overall diet delivers the necessary nutrients in the right proportions.

Achieving nutrient balance is crucial in ration formulation. This involves meticulous calculation and adjustment to ensure that the diet provides optimal levels of each nutrient required by the cattle. Overlooking any essential nutrient can lead to deficiencies or imbalances, potentially impacting growth, reproduction, and overall herd health.

Optimizing feed efficiency is another key goal. Efficient diets not only meet nutritional requirements but also minimize waste and maximize feed utilization. This approach not only enhances profitability by reducing feed costs but also promotes sustainability by minimizing environmental impact associated with feed production and waste management.

Successful ration formulation demands a comprehensive knowledge of feed composition and cattle nutritional requirements. Nutritionists must stay informed about the nutrient content of various feedstuffs and understand how these nutrients interact within the digestive system of cattle. This knowledge forms the basis for making informed decisions that align with production goals and economic constraints.

In practice, ration formulation involves iterative adjustments based on ongoing evaluation of cattle performance and changing environmental conditions. Periodic assessments ensure that diets remain optimized for current needs and are adjusted as cattle progress through different production stages.

Ultimately, the goal of ration formulation is to support the overall well-being of beef cattle while maximizing productivity and efficiency. By adhering to these principles—understanding nutrient requirements, selecting appropriate feed ingredients, balancing nutrients, and optimizing feed efficiency—nutritionists play a pivotal role in the success and sustainability of beef cattle operations. Through careful planning and continuous refinement, producers can ensure that their cattle receive diets that promote health, growth, and reproductive success, ultimately contributing to the profitability and long-term viability of their operations.

BALANCING RATIONS FOR NUTRIENT NEEDS

Balancing rations for livestock involves a meticulous process aimed at ensuring animals receive optimal nutrition tailored to their specific needs. This practice is crucial for maintaining health, supporting growth, and maximizing production efficiency. The process typically involves several key steps that collectively contribute to formulating well-balanced diets.

Nutrient Analysis:

The first step in balancing rations is conducting a thorough nutrient analysis of various feed ingredients. This can be achieved through laboratory testing to accurately measure the nutrient composition of each feedstuff. Alternatively, standard values from established feed composition tables are utilized, providing baseline nutrient content information. This analysis encompasses critical nutrients such as energy, protein, fiber, vitamins, and minerals, which are essential for animal growth, reproduction, and overall health.

Calculating Requirements:

Once the nutrient content of feed ingredients is determined, the next step involves calculating the specific nutritional requirements of the livestock being fed. These requirements vary depending on factors such as the animal's species, age, weight, physiological state (e.g., lactation, gestation), and intended use (e.g., growth, maintenance, reproduction). Nutritional requirements are typically expressed as daily or periodic needs for energy (calories), protein (amino acids), minerals (calcium, phosphorus, etc.), and vitamins essential for metabolic processes and bodily functions.

Formulating Diets:

With both the nutrient content of feedstuffs and the nutritional requirements of the animals at hand, the formulation of balanced diets begins. This step involves combining different feed ingredients in precise ratios to achieve the desired levels of nutrients in the diet. The goal is to meet or exceed the animal's requirements without oversupplying nutrients, which could be wasteful and costly. Factors such as the digestibility of feedstuffs and the bioavailability of nutrients are also considered to ensure that animals can efficiently utilize the nutrients provided.

Adjusting for Specific Goals:

Formulating diets is not a one-size-fits-all approach. Depending on the specific production goals, adjustments may be necessary. For instance, diets may need to be formulated to support higher growth rates in young animals, increased milk production in lactating cows, or optimal body condition in breeding stock. This customization involves fine-tuning the proportions of different feed ingredients to optimize nutrient intake relative to the animal's performance objectives.

Monitoring and Evaluation:

After formulating diets, ongoing monitoring and evaluation are essential to ensure that the nutritional needs of the animals are consistently met. This includes periodically reassessing feed ingredients' nutrient content, adjusting diets based on changes in animal requirements (e.g., growth stages), and evaluating the animals' overall health and performance. Feedback from production records and veterinary assessments helps refine feeding programs to achieve optimal results.

FEED MIXING AND DELIVERY METHODS

In modern livestock management, ensuring cattle receive balanced nutrition is pivotal for maintaining health and optimizing productivity. This process begins with precise feed formulation and extends to meticulous feed mixing and delivery methods that guarantee every animal receives adequate nutrition.

Feed mixing is a critical stage where various feed ingredients are combined to create a homogeneous blend. This ensures that each mouthful consumed by the cattle provides a balanced array of nutrients. Given the diverse nature of feed ingredients—varying in densities, particle sizes, and nutritional compositions—proper mixing is essential to prevent segregation and ensure uniformity. This uniformity not only promotes optimal growth and performance but also supports digestive health by preventing selective eating, where animals may pick and choose preferred components, potentially leading to imbalances in their diet.

Delivery systems play an equally vital role in the feeding process. Choosing appropriate feeding systems, such as troughs, feed bunks, or automated feeders, depends on factors like herd size, feeding frequency, and the type of ration being administered. These systems are designed not only to provide easy access to feed but also to minimize waste. For instance, automated feeders can dispense precise amounts of feed at scheduled intervals, reducing overconsumption and ensuring that feed is always available without risk of spoilage.

Feeding frequency and timing are strategic considerations in optimizing feed intake and digestion. Regular feeding schedules help maintain consistent nutrient intake, which is crucial for the animal's metabolic processes and overall health. Abrupt changes in feeding times or delays can lead to digestive disturbances and affect feed efficiency. Therefore, maintaining a reliable feeding routine supports the cattle's digestive function and enhances their ability to utilize nutrients effectively.

Quality control measures are integral throughout the entire feed management process. From ingredient sourcing to final feed delivery, monitoring and maintaining feed quality ensures consistency and prevents contamination or spoilage. Quality control protocols may include regular sampling and analysis of feed ingredients, checking for moisture levels and microbial contamination, and ensuring that storage conditions are optimal to preserve nutritional integrity.

Additionally, proper storage of feed ingredients and mixed rations is essential to prevent spoilage and maintain freshness. Improperly stored feed can lead to nutrient degradation and the growth of molds or toxins, which pose health risks to livestock if consumed.

MONITORING AND ADJUSTING FEEDING PROGRAMS

Monitoring and adjusting feeding programs for cattle is a critical component of ensuring optimal performance and health. By closely observing several key factors, farmers can effectively manage their herds' nutritional needs and adapt to changing conditions.

Feed Intake Monitoring: One of the primary tasks in managing cattle nutrition is monitoring daily feed intake. This involves ensuring that each animal consumes the expected amount of nutrients based on their stage of growth or production. Deviations in intake can serve as early indicators of various issues. For instance, a decrease in feed consumption might signal health problems, such as illness or stress, or indicate issues with feed palatability. Conversely, an increase in intake might suggest a need for adjustments in the ration formulation to meet the animals' nutritional requirements adequately.

Body Condition Assessment: Regular assessment of body condition scores (BCS) is essential for evaluating the nutritional status of cattle. BCS provides valuable insights into whether animals are receiving sufficient nutrition to support their health and reproductive capabilities. Maintaining optimal body condition is crucial for reproductive success, milk production in dairy cows, and overall herd health. Based on BCS evaluations, farmers can adjust feeding levels to ensure cattle remain in optimal condition throughout different stages of their lifecycle.

Performance Metrics Tracking: Tracking performance metrics such as growth rates, milk production (for lactating cows), and reproductive performance is fundamental to evaluating the effectiveness of feeding programs. These metrics provide quantitative data on how well the current feeding regimen supports the desired production goals. For example, if growth rates are below expectations or milk production levels are declining, adjustments to the feeding program may be necessary. This could involve modifying the types or quantities of feed provided to better meet the nutritional needs of the cattle and enhance their performance.

Environmental Considerations: Environmental factors play a significant role in cattle nutrition and must be taken into account when designing feeding programs. Factors such as temperature extremes, humidity levels, and seasonal changes can impact feed intake and nutrient requirements. During hot weather, for instance, cattle may consume less feed due to heat stress, necessitating adjustments in feeding strategies to ensure adequate nutrient intake. Similarly, cold temperatures can increase energy requirements as animals expend more energy to maintain body temperature, requiring adjustments in feed formulations to meet these increased energy needs.

Adaptation and Optimization: The process of monitoring and adjusting feeding programs is not static but rather dynamic and ongoing. It involves continual observation, data collection, and analysis to identify trends or deviations that may require intervention. By staying vigilant and responsive to changes in feed intake, body condition, performance metrics, and environmental conditions, farmers can optimize their feeding programs to maximize cattle health, productivity, and overall profitability.

CHAPTER SIX

HEALTH AND NUTRITION INTERACTIONS

NUTRITIONAL DISORDERS AND DEFICIENCIES

Nutritional disorders and deficiencies profoundly affect the health, growth, and productivity of beef cattle. These conditions arise primarily from inadequate intake or imbalances of essential nutrients critical for bodily functions. Among the most prevalent are mineral deficiencies, vitamin deficiencies, and protein-energy malnutrition.

Mineral deficiencies pose significant risks to cattle health. Essential minerals such as calcium, phosphorus, magnesium, zinc, and selenium play pivotal roles in metabolic processes and immune function. Insufficient intake of calcium can lead to hypocalcemia, commonly known as milk fever, particularly problematic during calving when demand for calcium spikes. Phosphorus deficiency results in poor bone development and reproductive issues, impacting overall herd fertility. Magnesium deficiency can cause grass tetany, characterized by nervous system disturbances in grazing cattle. Trace minerals like zinc and selenium are crucial for immune response; their deficiency weakens cattle defenses against diseases.

Vitamin deficiencies also contribute to numerous health issues in beef cattle.

Vitamins A, D, E, and various B-complex vitamins are indispensable for growth, reproduction, immune function, and overall vitality. Vitamin A deficiency can lead to vision problems, impaired growth, and susceptibility to infections. Vitamin D deficiency results in poor calcium absorption and skeletal deformities. Vitamin E deficiency increases the risk of muscular disorders and reproductive inefficiencies. B-complex vitamins are essential for energy metabolism and nerve function; their scarcity can hinder growth rates and weaken immune defenses.

Protein-energy malnutrition arises when cattle fail to consume adequate protein and/or energy for their metabolic needs.

This deficiency manifests in reduced growth rates, diminished milk production in lactating cows, and compromised immune responses. Insufficient protein intake limits muscle development and milk yield, impacting both animal welfare and economic returns for cattle producers. Energy deficits exacerbate these effects, as they are crucial for maintaining body condition and supporting physiological processes.

Management strategies to mitigate these nutritional challenges include balanced feed formulations tailored to specific herd requirements, supplemented with minerals, vitamins, and protein sources as needed. Monitoring feed quality and ensuring access to fresh, nutritious forage are critical practices. Regular health assessments and diagnostic testing can detect early signs of deficiencies, enabling prompt intervention through dietary adjustments or targeted supplementation.

Effective nutrition management not only promotes cattle health and productivity but also supports sustainable farming practices. Addressing nutritional disorders promptly enhances animal welfare, reduces veterinary costs, and optimizes overall farm profitability. Educating livestock caretakers about the importance of balanced nutrition and preventive measures is crucial for maintaining robust cattle herds capable of thriving in various environmental conditions.

ROLE OF NUTRITION IN DISEASE PREVENTION

Nutrition plays a pivotal role in safeguarding the health and preventing diseases in beef cattle. A properly balanced diet is not merely about fulfilling nutritional requirements but is crucial in supporting various physiological functions that collectively enhance the resilience of cattle against diseases.

Firstly, the immune system of beef cattle heavily relies on a spectrum of essential nutrients. Vitamins such as A, D, E, and C are instrumental in bolstering immune responses. For instance, Vitamin A plays a vital role in maintaining epithelial integrity, which serves as the first line of defense against pathogens. Vitamin D supports immune function through its regulatory effects on immune cells. Vitamin E is a potent antioxidant that protects cell membranes from oxidative damage, thereby promoting robust immune responses. Additionally, minerals like zinc, copper, and selenium are indispensable for enzymatic reactions and antioxidant defenses within immune cells, ensuring their optimal functioning. A well-nourished immune system is better equipped to fend off infectious diseases, thereby reducing disease incidence among cattle herds.

Secondly, the maintenance of gut health is intricately linked to a balanced diet in beef cattle. The rumen, the largest compartment of the stomach, houses a diverse population of microorganisms crucial for the fermentation and digestion of feed. A balanced diet promotes a healthy rumen environment, ensuring an optimal microbial population and fermentation process. This, in turn, supports efficient digestion and absorption of nutrients, minimizing the risk of digestive disorders such as acidosis and bloat. Acidosis, for instance, can occur when there is an imbalance in rumen pH due to excessive intake of readily fermentable carbohydrates. A diet carefully balanced with appropriate fiber content and fermentable carbohydrates helps maintain rumen health, thereby reducing the likelihood of digestive disturbances.

Furthermore, bone and muscle health are vital considerations in beef cattle nutrition. Adequate levels of calcium, phosphorus, and vitamin D are essential for skeletal development, bone mineralization, and muscle function. Calcium and phosphorus are structural components of bones, while vitamin D facilitates their absorption and utilization. Strong bones and muscles not only contribute to the overall structural integrity of cattle but also reduce the incidence of injuries and lameness, thereby promoting animal welfare and productivity.

MANAGING STRESS THROUGH NUTRITION

Managing stress in beef cattle is crucial for maintaining their health and optimizing productivity across various conditions, including weaning, transportation, and extreme weather events. Nutrition plays a pivotal role in mitigating the detrimental effects of stress, offering essential support through energy provision, electrolyte balance maintenance, and the incorporation of adaptogens.

One of the primary ways nutrition supports stressed cattle is through energy provision. During stressful periods such as weaning or transportation, cattle experience heightened metabolic demands. Diets enriched with high-energy ingredients like grains or fats provide the necessary calories to meet these increased energy needs. Adequate energy intake not only sustains basic bodily functions but also helps in maintaining optimal growth rates and supports immune function, which can otherwise be compromised under stress.

Electrolyte balance is another critical aspect influenced by nutrition during stress management. Proper electrolyte levels, including sodium, potassium, and chloride, are essential for maintaining cellular function and regulating fluid balance. During stressful situations, such as hot weather or transportation, cattle are prone to dehydration due to increased water loss through sweat or respiratory evaporation. Diets formulated with balanced electrolytes help prevent dehydration and maintain physiological homeostasis, thereby supporting overall health and performance.

Incorporating adaptogens into cattle diets is a strategic approach to enhancing stress resilience. Adaptogens are nutrients or herbal supplements known for their ability to help organisms adapt to stressors more efficiently. For instance, vitamins like vitamin C act as antioxidants, mitigating oxidative stress induced by transportation or changes in diet. Selenium is another crucial nutrient that supports immune function and protects against oxidative damage, contributing to overall stress management in cattle. Additionally, adaptogenic herbs such as certain plant extracts have shown promise in reducing stress-related symptoms and supporting immune responses in livestock.

The synergistic effects of these nutritional strategies are evident in their collective ability to bolster cattle health and productivity during stressful events.

By optimizing energy intake, maintaining electrolyte balance, and leveraging adaptogenic properties, producers can mitigate the negative impacts of stress on beef cattle. This proactive approach not only enhances animal welfare but also supports sustainable production practices by reducing the incidence of stress-related illnesses and improving overall herd resilience.

Furthermore, tailoring nutrition to specific stressors allows for targeted interventions that align with the unique challenges faced by cattle in various production environments. For example, adjusting feed formulations during periods of extreme heat or cold can help cattle better cope with environmental stressors, minimizing performance losses and ensuring consistent growth rates.

USE OF PROBIOTICS AND PREBIOTICS

Probiotics and prebiotics play crucial roles in enhancing the health and productivity of beef cattle by promoting optimal gut function and overall well-being. These substances are integral components of modern livestock management, offering benefits that extend beyond basic nutrition to include improved digestion, nutrient absorption, and immune system support.

Probiotics are live microorganisms, such as bacteria and yeast, that confer health benefits when consumed in adequate quantities. In beef cattle, probiotics are particularly beneficial for maintaining a balanced microbial environment within the rumen. The rumen, a large fermentation chamber where fibrous plant material is broken down, relies on a complex ecosystem of microorganisms to efficiently digest feed. Probiotics help to enhance this process by introducing or supplementing beneficial microbes. These microbes aid in breaking down fibers that cattle typically consume, such as hay and grass, into nutrients that can be absorbed and utilized by the animal. By improving fiber digestion, probiotics contribute to increased feed efficiency and overall nutrient availability, thereby supporting the animal's growth and performance.

Moreover, probiotics play a significant role in mitigating digestive disorders in cattle, such as acidosis or bloat, which can occur due to dietary imbalances or stress. By promoting a stable microbial population in the rumen, probiotics help maintain pH balance and prevent harmful bacteria from proliferating. This not only improves digestive health but also reduces the incidence of metabolic disorders, ultimately leading to healthier and more resilient cattle.

Prebiotics, on the other hand, are non-digestible fibers that serve as food sources for beneficial bacteria already present in the gut. These fibers are not broken down by the animal's digestive enzymes but instead reach the lower gastrointestinal tract where they selectively stimulate the growth and activity of beneficial bacteria. By fostering the growth of these beneficial microbes, prebiotics contribute to a healthier gut environment and improve nutrient utilization efficiency. This means that cattle can derive more energy and nutrients from their feed, leading to improved growth rates and overall performance.

Additionally, prebiotics have been shown to enhance immune function in cattle. A healthy gut microbiota is closely linked to a robust immune response, as beneficial bacteria help to regulate immune system activity and defend against pathogens. By supporting the growth of beneficial bacteria, prebiotics indirectly bolster the animal's immune defenses, making them more resilient to infections and diseases.

In practical terms, the incorporation of probiotics and prebiotics into beef cattle diets is typically achieved through specially formulated feed additives or supplements. These products are designed to deliver precise amounts of beneficial microorganisms or prebiotic fibers to ensure optimal effectiveness. Farmers and ranchers often work closely with nutritionists and veterinarians to determine the most suitable probiotic and prebiotic formulations based on their herd's specific nutritional needs and health considerations.

CHAPTER SEVEN

ECONOMIC AND ENVIRONMENTAL CONSIDERATIONS

COST-EFFECTIVE FEEDING STRATEGIES

Cost-effective feeding strategies play a crucial role in optimizing productivity and minimizing costs in beef cattle production. These strategies encompass various approaches aimed at enhancing feed efficiency while maintaining or improving the overall health and performance of the cattle.

Ration Formulation is a foundational aspect of cost-effective feeding. It involves carefully balancing the nutritional requirements of the cattle with the cost-effective selection of feed ingredients and supplements. The goal is to create diets that not only meet the nutritional needs of the cattle but also do so efficiently. This process often involves utilizing a mix of grains, forages, protein supplements, and minerals in proportions that maximize digestibility and utilization by the cattle.

Feed Management practices are essential for reducing waste and optimizing feed utilization. Proper storage of feed to maintain freshness and nutritional quality is critical. This includes protecting feed from pests, moisture, and exposure to elements that could degrade its quality. Handling practices ensure that feed is not wasted during transfer and feeding, thereby maximizing the amount of feed that is actually consumed by the cattle. Efficient feeding methods, such as using feeders that minimize spillage and spoilage, further contribute to cost savings and improved efficiency.

Alternative Feedstuffs offer opportunities to reduce feed costs by incorporating by-products and non-traditional feed sources that provide nutritional benefits at a lower cost compared to conventional feeds. Examples include distillers grains from ethanol production, soybean hulls, and bakery waste. These alternative feedstuffs can be used to partially replace more expensive components of the diet without compromising nutritional quality, thereby reducing overall feeding costs.

Grazing Management is another crucial strategy in cost-effective feeding, particularly for operations with access to pasture and forage resources. Rotational grazing systems allow for efficient utilization of available pasture by moving cattle between different grazing areas. This approach not only improves forage utilization but also promotes regrowth and reduces the need for supplemental feeds. By minimizing reliance on purchased feeds, grazing management contributes significantly to lowering overall feeding costs.

Implementing these strategies requires careful monitoring and adjustment based on factors such as cattle growth stage, environmental conditions, and market prices of feed ingredients. Regular assessment of feed efficiency metrics, such as feed conversion ratios and cost per unit of gain, helps producers evaluate the effectiveness of their feeding strategies and identify areas for improvement.

EVALUATING FEED COSTS AND RETURNS

Evaluating feed costs and returns is crucial for optimizing the economic efficiency of feeding programs in livestock management, particularly in the context of cattle production. This evaluation involves several key considerations that directly impact profitability and operational decision-making.

Firstly, feed efficiency is a fundamental metric in assessing the productivity of feeding programs. This is typically quantified through the calculation of feed conversion ratios (FCR), which measure how effectively cattle convert feed into meat. A lower FCR indicates higher efficiency, as less feed is required to produce a unit of meat. Monitoring and improving FCR is essential for reducing feed costs and enhancing overall profitability.

Another critical factor in evaluating feed costs and returns is the cost-per-unit of gain. This metric involves comparing the cost of feed per pound of weight gain achieved by the cattle. By optimizing feeding programs to achieve the lowest possible cost-per-unit of gain, ranchers can maximize profitability. This optimization often involves balancing the nutritional needs of the cattle with cost-effective feed options to achieve optimal growth rates.

Feed price variability is another significant consideration. The prices of essential feed components such as grains and supplements can fluctuate due to market conditions, weather patterns, and global demand. Ranchers must monitor these fluctuations closely and adjust their feeding strategies accordingly. For instance, during periods of high feed prices, alternative feed sources or ration adjustments may be considered to manage costs while maintaining cattle health and growth.

Market conditions play a pivotal role in the economic evaluation of feed costs and returns. Fluctuations in both beef prices and feed input prices directly influence profitability. Ranchers need to analyze market trends and forecasts to make informed decisions about when to buy feed, when to sell cattle, and how to adjust feeding programs to maximize returns on investment. Understanding market dynamics allows for strategic planning and risk management in cattle production.

Additionally, technological advancements and innovations in feed formulation and management practices can significantly impact feed costs and efficiency. Adopting modern feeding technologies, such as precision feeding systems and improved feed formulations, can enhance feed utilization efficiency and reduce overall costs.

Furthermore, sustainability considerations are increasingly important in feed cost evaluations. Efficient feeding practices not only improve economic outcomes but also reduce environmental impacts by minimizing resource use and waste production.

ENVIRONMENTAL IMPACT OF BEEF CATTLE NUTRITION

Beef cattle nutrition plays a crucial role in shaping environmental sustainability, necessitating thoughtful management and strategies to mitigate its ecological footprint across various fronts.

Resource Use

Efficient management of resources is pivotal in beef cattle nutrition. Water, a precious resource, is utilized extensively in both feed production and cattle consumption. Growing feed crops demands substantial irrigation, contributing to agricultural water stress in regions where water availability is limited. Moreover, grazing lands require careful stewardship to prevent degradation and ensure sustainable use.

Balancing the water needs between crop irrigation and cattle hydration is essential to minimize water scarcity impacts associated with beef cattle nutrition.

Land use is another critical consideration. Grazing lands must be managed to maintain their productivity and ecological integrity. Simultaneously, cultivating feed crops necessitates arable land, which can lead to deforestation or habitat loss if not managed sustainably. Responsible land use practices, such as rotational grazing and agroforestry, can mitigate environmental impacts by enhancing soil health, biodiversity, and carbon sequestration potential.

Greenhouse Gas Emissions

Greenhouse gas (GHG) emissions from beef cattle nutrition are primarily attributed to methane from enteric fermentation and carbon dioxide from feed production and transportation. Methane, a potent GHG, is produced during digestion in the cattle's rumen. Strategies like improved feed efficiency, dietary adjustments, and methane-reducing additives are being explored to mitigate these emissions. Additionally, optimizing feed sourcing and transport logistics can reduce the carbon footprint associated with feed production, further contributing to GHG emission reductions.

Nutrient Management

Nutrient management is crucial to safeguarding water quality and ecosystem health. Manure from beef cattle contains nitrogen and phosphorus, which can leach into water bodies, causing eutrophication and harming aquatic ecosystems. Moreover, fertilizers used in feed crop cultivation can contribute to nutrient runoff if not applied judiciously. Implementing best management practices such as precision agriculture, nutrient cycling, and controlled application of manure and fertilizers can minimize nutrient losses, preserve soil fertility, and protect water quality.

Integrated Approaches

Addressing the environmental impacts of beef cattle nutrition requires integrated approaches that consider the interconnectedness of water, land, and air quality. Sustainable intensification practices, such as integrating livestock with crop production systems (e.g., agroecology), can optimize resource use efficiency while minimizing environmental degradation. Utilizing innovative technologies like precision agriculture, advanced feed formulations, and methane mitigation strategies can further enhance sustainability efforts in beef cattle nutrition.

SUSTAINABLE FEEDING PRACTICES

Sustainable feeding practices in beef cattle nutrition are crucial for balancing economic profitability with environmental stewardship and social responsibility. These practices aim to optimize resource use, minimize environmental impact, and ensure long-term viability of cattle farming.

Efficient resource use lies at the heart of sustainable feeding practices. By carefully selecting and managing feed ingredients, farmers can reduce waste and enhance efficiency. This approach not only lowers production costs but also lessens the ecological footprint of beef production. Efficient resource use encompasses choosing feed ingredients that are locally available and environmentally sustainable. For example, using locally grown crops reduces transportation emissions and supports regional agricultural economies.

Conservation practices play a pivotal role in sustainable beef cattle nutrition. Soil conservation measures such as rotational grazing and minimal tillage help maintain soil health and productivity. Healthy soils support robust pasture growth, which in turn sustains cattle nutrition without excessive reliance on artificial inputs. Water management strategies are equally vital, ensuring that water resources are utilized responsibly and efficiently across grazing lands. Implementing biodiversity conservation measures further enhances the ecological balance of these landscapes, promoting habitats for native species and preserving natural ecosystems.

The exploration and utilization of alternative feeds and by-products are central to sustainable feeding practices. By diversifying feed sources beyond traditional grains and forages, farmers can reduce dependency on finite resources. Utilizing by-products from food processing industries not only reduces waste but also provides nutritious supplements for cattle diets. This approach contributes to resource efficiency by recycling nutrients back into the food production cycle, thus minimizing environmental impact.

Reducing the carbon footprint of beef cattle production is another critical objective of sustainable feeding practices. Adopting technologies and management practices that mitigate greenhouse gas emissions is essential. For instance, optimizing feed formulations to minimize methane emissions from enteric fermentation in cattle can significantly lower the overall carbon intensity of beef production. Additionally, enhancing carbon sequestration through practices like agroforestry or pasture management contributes to offsetting emissions, thereby promoting a more sustainable carbon balance.

Educational initiatives and collaborative efforts among stakeholders are integral to advancing sustainable feeding practices in beef cattle nutrition. Farmers benefit from access to research-backed information and practical guidelines for implementing these practices on their operations. Government support and industry partnerships play pivotal roles in facilitating the adoption of sustainable practices through policy incentives, research funding, and market opportunities for sustainably produced beef.

THE END

www.ingramcontent.com/pod-product-compliance
Lightning Source LLC
Chambersburg PA
CBHW071831210526
45479CB00001B/81